A Parent's Guide to Overcoming Picky Eating in Children

Unlocking the Joy of Eating

Jessica W. Brown

Copyright © Jessica W. Brown, 2024.

Disclaimer

The information provided in this book is for general informational purposes only. While every effort has been made to ensure the accuracy of the information contained within this book, the author and publisher assume no responsibility for errors or omissions, or for damages resulting from the use of the information contained herein.

This book is sold with the understanding that the author and publisher are not engaged in rendering legal, financial, medical, or other professional advice. The reader should consult with a professional in the respective field for any such advice.

Table Of Contents

CHAPTER 1

Picky Eating In Children

Picky eating (also known as fussy, faddy, or choosy eating) is typically classed as one of a variety of feeding issues. It is distinguished by an inability to eat familiar meals or to try new foods, as well as strong dietary preferences.

Picky eating is quite prevalent among children. It often begins in the toddler years, peaks around three years old, and then fades by the time the child reaches five. Parents are very concerned about what their children eat (or do not consume). However, most children get enough nourishment from their meals throughout the week.

Your child may be picky about what he or she eats for a variety of reasons, including a sensitivity to smells, tastes, or textures. It's also likely that your youngster has underlying sensory issues or eating habits shaped by punishments and rewards. As we progress, we will look at some of the symptoms, causes, and other aspects of picky eating.

How Can I Tell If My Child Is a Picky Eater?

If your child is a fussy eater, look for the following signs:

You force-feed your child. You and your family find mealtimes difficult. It takes around 30 minutes to finish a meal. Your child will not eat certain foods, such as veggies, meats, or foods with a specific texture. Your child will only eat when watching movies, programs, television, or other kinds of entertainment.

He or she will only consume a modest assortment of food with varied flavors and textures, indicating that they only eat less than 20 types of food. At 16 to 18 months old, your child is still consuming the majority of baby foods. After 12 months, your child is having trouble transitioning from milk to semi-solid foods. **Refuses to try new kinds of foods.**

Causes of Picky Eating

Picky eating can be caused by early feeding issues, the late introduction of lumpy foods during weaning, pressure to eat, and early food selectivity, particularly if the mother is concerned. Fresh food and having the same meal with your child can help prevent picky eating.

Like adults, children have a favorite food. Whether it's bread with jam or homemade spaghetti, your youngster will develop a taste. However, even if your children are free to eat anything they want, you should still keep an eye on their diet. Over time, your child may acquire unhealthy eating patterns and food choices. While occasional indulgence is permissible, neglecting their nutrition might hurt their overall health.

To keep mealtime from becoming a battle, you must understand why children become picky eaters and what you can do to help them overcome it.

Understanding the typical causes of selective eating is critical for parents. These causes can be broadly categorized into five groups, providing insights into the elements that contribute to selective eating habits.

Parents should be aware that, in some situations, a child's refusal to consume specific foods may be due to medical difficulties. If you suspect any of these problems, you should see a doctor.

Here are the common reasons for finicky eating:

1. High sugar consumption. Excessive artificial sugar consumption is the most effective approach to transform your youngster into a fussy eater. Sweetened juice, cookies, candy, and other similar snacks consumed too frequently will condition their taste for sweets, impacting their appetite at mealtimes. Setting appropriate limitations will assist you in resolving this issue while avoiding additional health complications.

2. Incorrectly cooked food. Before you begin setting the table, double-check the dish you are cooking. Serving badly cooked food, whether rotten or raw, can be quite uncomfortable for your child. Always keep in mind that youngsters associate meals with certain experiences. If people eat a poorly prepared version of a specific meal, they may recall the unpleasant taste or experience, preventing them from eating it again.

3. Inconsistent mealtimes Sticking to a routine will help keep your children's appetites regular. Serving food at irregular intervals will produce fluctuations in their hunger levels, prompting them to nibble excessively. Because they don't know when the appropriate mealtimes are, they may snack shortly before lunch or supper. Setting a specific timetable for breakfast, lunch, and dinner is an easy solution to this.

4. Power struggle. If your child refuses the meal you provide, do not force them to eat it. Using your parental power may communicate the wrong message, which can have a variety of consequences. They will establish a bad association with a meal, which may have an impact on their relationship with you. Unfortunately, many parents may resort to bribing their children with dessert or preparing another meal to get them to eat—this technique promotes fussy eating and may eventually exacerbate the condition.

5. They are genetically sensitive to certain foods. Genetics can influence dietary preferences. A study of youngsters aged 5 to 10 discovered that those who were more sensitive to bitter-tasting chemicals preferred sweeter foods. When planning a dinner, keep in mind that your child may not have the same taste preferences as you do. Experimenting with different flavors and speaking with your child will help you identify the best flavors for their taste buds.

Furthermore, children's eating preferences can alter dramatically over time. Your child may dislike a certain flavor at first and then come to enjoy it later. Do not be afraid to return certain elements and flavors at a later date, possibly prepared slightly differently.

Signs of Picky Eating: When to Worry?

It is perfectly typical for youngsters to demonstrate some degree of finicky eating behavior during their early years.

However, it is also crucial for parents to remain watchful and identify when these eating habits suggest a more serious problem.

Persistent refusal of whole food groups: A regular rejection of entire food groups, such as fruits and vegetables, can be cause for concern because it may result in nutritional inadequacies.

Dramatic weight reduction or stagnation: A big decline in your child's weight or a plateau in their growth are two of the more obvious indicators of a picky eating problem.

Emotional Distress: If your child is experiencing emotional distress, tantrums, or anxiety during mealtimes, it may indicate that their connection with food is becoming troublesome.

Gagging, spitting, and swallowing issues: If your child frequently has difficulties swallowing, gagging, or spitting while trying new meals, this may indicate sensory or physical concerns with eating that need to be addressed.

If you notice several of these symptoms in your child's fussy eating behavior, consult a healthcare practitioner. Remember that early intervention can significantly improve your child's general health and well-being.

Tips for Parents of Picky Eaters

Here are some tips for parents with finicky eaters:

Remain calm and patient: Dealing with a finicky eater can be irritating, but it's critical to stay calm and patient. Avoid turning mealtime into a war, as this can exacerbate the situation.

Respect their preferences. Forcing people to eat items they detest can result in unfavorable associations with those foods. Try waiting for your child's appetite to develop. If they opt not to eat lunch, there is a good possibility they will be more interested in the dinner you've cooked.

Provide a positive example: Children often copy their parents' actions. If they witness you enjoying a variety of meals, they will be more willing to try them themselves.

Provide a diverse range of foods: Try to introduce foods from several food groups. Eat fruits, veggies, lean proteins, and whole grains. This exposure may help broaden their palate over time.

Provide nourishment with fewer sugars. Don't forget to check your powdered milk drink to ensure that it provides nourishment while also being low in sugar. Choose one without added artificial sugars. Stick to a regimen.

Attempt to establish a consistent eating pattern. Children frequently feel more safe when they know when their meals will arrive. Make meals enjoyable. Create a pleasant and relaxing mealtime environment by removing distractions such as electronics and focusing on enjoying the meal together as a family.

Consult a professional. If you're concerned about your child's nutrition or finicky eating habits, go to a pediatrician, registered dietitian, or feeding specialist for advice and assistance.

Remember that fussy eating is a normal phase for many youngsters and usually improves with time. However, if you are concerned about your child's growth, health, or the severity of their picky eating, get professional advice to ensure they are receiving the nutrients they require for development.

What You Should Not Do

Mealtimes can be challenging if your child is a picky eater, and you may unintentionally compound the situation.

Here are some things you shouldn't do:

Forced feeding Force feeding can be distressing for both you and your child, and it may cause your child to develop bad feelings and mental states linked with eating.

Give your youngster sugary drinks or snacks an hour before dinner. These may reduce the child's appetite.

Inquiring as to whether he or she enjoys or dislikes the new food you have served them. Instead, discuss the shape, color, and flavor of the dish to pique their interest and engagement.

Threaten or reprimand your youngster if he or she doesn't eat. Instead, remain calm and neutral.

Do not push him/her to eat it while maintaining your firm stance on unacceptable behaviors (for example, throwing food, or shouting).

CHAPTER 2

Promoting Healthy Eating Habits In Children

Childhood is a critical period for the development of lifelong habits, particularly those related to eating and nutrition. Nurturing healthy eating habits in children is critical not only for their growth and development but also for avoiding the beginning of chronic disorders in adulthood. In an age where fast food and sugary snacks are easily accessible, it is more vital than ever for parents and caregivers to play an active part in fostering healthy eating habits.

This section discusses the importance of instilling good eating habits in youngsters and offers practical advice on how to accomplish this objective.

The Value of Healthy Eating Habits in Children's

Physical Health. Physical health is strongly linked to proper food choices in children. A well-balanced diet provides the nutrients needed for proper development, growth, and overall health. Proper nutrition aids youngsters in maintaining a healthy weight, developing strong bones and muscles, and supporting the proper function of their vital organs.

Cognitive Development. Nutrition plays a vital role in cognitive development. Children who eat a diet rich in critical nutrients do better in school and solve problems. Certain nutrients, such as omega-3 fatty acids, are essential for brain development, as well as improved memory and concentration.

Emotional and Behavioral Well-being. Eating habits might affect a child's emotional and behavioral well-being. A diet heavy in sugar and processed foods can cause mood swings and hyperactivity, sometimes known as the "sugar rush." On the other side, a diet high in grains, fruits, and vegetables can help to stabilize mood and enhance behavior.

Long-Term Wellness. Children who adopt healthy eating habits are more likely to keep them into adulthood. This not only minimizes the risk of juvenile obesity, but also greatly lowers the likelihood of developing chronic health disorders such as diabetes, heart disease, and hypertension later in life. Thus, habits developed during childhood act as an effective preventive measure.

Tips for promoting healthy eating habits

It is critical to recognize that a child's early years often build the framework for their future nutritional choices. Children should be introduced to nutritious foods and healthy eating habits.

Here are some healthy dietary suggestions for kids:

Lead by example. Children frequently replicate adult behavior, therefore parents and caregivers must serve as role models for good eating. If youngsters see adults eating a range of nutritious foods, they are more likely to follow suit. Make mealtimes a pleasant and communal affair, promoting the notion that nutritious food is both delicious and fun.

Create a Positive Food Environment. A favorable food environment can lead to healthier eating habits. Keep nutritious snacks easily available in the house and limit your intake of sugary and processed foods. Make fruits, veggies, and whole grains the highlight of your cupboard and refrigerator.

Involve children in meal preparation. Engaging youngsters in meal preparation can be an enjoyable learning opportunity. Allow kids to take part in age-appropriate cooking duties like washing vegetables, stirring, or preparing the table. When children help prepare their meals, they are more likely to try new foods and get a sense of control over their dietary choices.

Offer a variety of foods. Introducing toddlers to a wide range of meals at an early age will help them develop a taste for different flavors and textures. Encourage them to try new fruits, vegetables, and proteins. Experiment with different cooking methods to create appetizing dishes.

Portion Control. Proper portion control is essential for keeping a healthy weight. Serve age-appropriate portions and avoid the 'clean your plate' approach, which can lead to overeating. Encourage youngsters to listen to their bodies and eat until they are full, not just until their plate is empty.

Limit sugary and processed foods. While it is acceptable to indulge in treats on occasion, sugary and processed foods should be limited in a child's diet. These foods are frequently lacking in nutritional value, which can lead to weight gain and other health problems. Save sugary snacks for special occasions and replace everyday soda with water or a healthier option.

Establish regular meal times. Consistent meal times provide a feeling of habit and structure for youngsters, allowing them to anticipate when they will be fed. Avoid skipping meals, particularly breakfast, which is vital for energy and attention. Make mealtimes a family event whenever possible.

Encourage water consumption. Water is essential for good hydration and general well-being. Encourage your children to drink plenty of water throughout the day, especially in between meals. Sugary beverages, such as soda and excessive fruit juices, should be avoided because they can lead to weight gain and tooth problems.

Be patient and flexible. Healthy eating habits in youngsters can be developed gradually. It is critical to be patient and adaptable because youngsters may be hesitant to sample new foods or go through stages of dietary preferences. Instead of forcing them into eating something they loathe, suggest alternatives.

Educate about nutrition. As children grow, teach them the value of nutrition and the benefits of a healthy diet. Teach kids how to read food labels and make informed decisions. Provide age-appropriate information on the nutritional worth of various foods.

Instilling healthy eating habits in children is an investment in their future well-being. Parents and caregivers can assist their children in establishing a lifelong knowledge of healthy eating by creating a positive food environment, acting as role models, and providing a variety of nutritious meals. These efforts will help a child's physical health, cognitive development, emotional well-being, and general quality of life.

CHAPTER 3

Children's Eating Preferences

Children frequently acquire food preferences throughout their childhood. However, some youngsters will refuse to consume a wide range of foods and have "definite food preferences". The following information will help you identify the "resistant eater" as a parent, teacher, or early childhood professional, explain some possible causes of the problem, and make some suggestions for things you may try with your child.

Characteristics of children who have clear food preferences:

They consume no more than fifteen types of food. It can be as little as two or three sorts, such as hot dogs, yogurt, and chicken nuggets.

They consume meals from only one or three food groups. When new foods are offered to them, they grow nervous (and may even throw tantrums).

They consume the same food prepared in the same manner over an extended period.

They may have developmental disabilities and/or a medical condition, such as Autism Spectrum Disorder, Cerebral Palsy, Muscular Dystrophy, and so on.

Eating issues and food aversions can be caused or contributed to by the following factors:

Poor oral and motor skills. Children with trouble biting, chewing, or swallowing may have drooling and resistance to new foods. Selective eating and difficulties digesting food.

Note: For children with weak oral-motor abilities, it is critical to advise families to seek professional medical counsel before attempting any new feeding practices.

Environmental and behavioral factors: "Food Neophobia" refers to the dread of novel foods. Unstructured mealtime environment (e.g., varied timetables and settings, or distractions during mealtime) Cultural beliefs/family practices (e.g., the child who is forced to eat or is penalized for not eating; the child who is not supposed to investigate the food with his fingers; the child who is fed until late in the preschool years) developmental difficulties (e.g., lack of speech due to poor oral-motor development; repetitive behaviors linked with Autism Spectrum Disorder; and cognitive delays).

Sensory and motor-based factors: Sensory Processing Disorder occurs when the brain has difficulties processing sensory information received from various parts of the body and/or the environment.

What you can do to support a child's good eating habits:

The tips below may help you and your "resistant eater" overcome his food aversions. Remember that this process will take time, therefore you must be consistent in implementing the tactics over and over again.

Collaborate with other staff members and parents to support the child. You can begin gathering information by asking questions about the child's eating habits (what, when, where, and how long), health, medical history, allergies, and diagnoses. Then you'll be ready to create a plan with the family so that everyone can start working toward the same goals.

Review the goals frequently and alter them as needed. The family should contemplate seeing a dietitian and an occupational therapist. An occupational therapist can offer solutions for addressing poor oral-motor development and sensory difficulties that may be related to the child's eating disorder. The mealtime routine should be as predictable and constant as feasible. Prepare the youngster for any changes in the surroundings (for example, a field trip). You can tell the group when and where the lunch will be, read a story about picnics, or compose a short social story for the occasion. Make sure the youngster understands the mealtime expectations, and that they are appropriate for his developmental level. Establish and discuss mealtime guidelines with the group.

Follow through with these regulations. Model and teach good eating habits and skills. Praise the child for trying new foods. Food Selection Make a list of the foods the youngster eats, the foods he used to eat, and the foods he does not consume from each major food group. This will give you a better idea of the items to introduce or that are lacking in the child's diet. Introduce new foods one by one, at the same time every day.

Menu items should represent all food groups. Discuss the dishes on the menu (taste, texture, fragrance, color). Prepare healthful and appetizing dishes for children (such as fruit cocktails). Allow for a choice of two or three healthy options. Offer at least one favorite food per meal but with a minor variation in presentation. Go grocery shopping with the group and let the child choose the "new food" from a healthy selection.

Create a "Menu of the Day" with the kids. Discuss what dishes will be served at lunch (including the one chosen by the youngster). If possible, cook the meal (or at least a portion of it) alongside the children. Always provide tiny servings of the new cuisine (in child-sized bowls). Initially, the goal could be for the youngster to be exposed to the new meal and be able to control his behavior (no crying or tantrums) when it is placed on his plate.

You can begin by placing the new food close to the youngster but on a separate dish. When you notice evidence of acceptance (acclimatization to the new circumstances), place one to two scoops of the new meal immediately on the child's plate. Always assess the child's emotions and reward him for appropriate behavior.

Make and use a First-Then visual board. This board will visually direct the child to the meals that will be served for lunch. Include the new dish as the first option and your favorite food as the second option. The child should take at least one or two bites of the "first" food. When he achieves this, he can eat his favorite food. Introduce the First-Then visual board after you notice the youngster becoming more comfortable with the "new food" experiences outlined above.

Allow for sensory exploration of new foods through planned, pleasurable activities. Sensory exploration allows the youngster to gradually become acquainted with a new meal by looking at, touching, and smelling it, without the pressure of eating it. The youngster learns about the new meal through fun and engaging activities.

Here are some examples of sensory activities:

The sensory pack contains two to four new food items. Hot potato game with various foods (put the food in a dish and pass it around). Smell and guess (blindfold or eyes closed); try new and preferred dishes. Grow a garden. Use dry food components for the sensory bin, art, and cognitive exercises (e.g., counting and sorting).

Having a child with specific food preferences can be difficult. It will be vital to spend time getting to know the child and learning about his situation, thinking positively about changing the child's habits, and giving and taking the time for the changes to occur.

CHAPTER 4

Sensory Food Aversion: Strategies To Help Your Picky Eater

Sensory Food Aversion In this section, we will define sensory food aversion and discuss ten effective strategies for helping your finicky eater. Some youngsters will refuse a few items, while others will refuse the majority of foods. Then, some children only consume one or two brands of food. You may have tried to hide it in a different pack, but they still know.

Toddlers frequently exhibit picky eating, sometimes known as the neophobia (fear of new foods) stage. Some children outgrow neophobia, while others do not.

What is sensory processing? Sensory processing is the way the brain receives, processes, and responds to information from the senses.

There are eight senses.

Olfactory (smell).

Visual (sight).

Tactile (touch).

Auditory (sound).

gustatory (taste).

proprioception (position of the body)

Vestibular mobility, balance, and direction of the body.

Interoception refers to internal physical sensations. First, sensory information is transmitted to us by external or internal stimuli.

The sensory information is then processed. Next, the body/mind reacts to the stimulus. Some people receive an excessive amount of sensory information, whereas others sense an insufficient amount. Those who have sensory processing issues may struggle to remain calm and awake when their senses become overwhelmed. This condition is known as sensory modulation disorder (SMD).

Children with SMD struggle to respond adequately to environmental stimuli and may be sensory over-responsive (SOR) or sensory under-responsive (SUR). A youngster with SOR may experience a sensation more intensely than usual. SOR may lead a youngster to go into "fight or flight" mode in reaction to overstimulating situations or environments. A little can seem like a lot in youngsters with SOR. A youngster with SUR, on the other hand, is unaware of the sensory inputs in their environment and hence does not respond. SUR children may appear apathetic since they exhibit little to no interest or passion in reaction to many stimuli. Children with SUR may perceive a lot as a small amount. These kids are generally sloppy eaters. This sensory processing problem can also affect a child's eating habits, which may manifest as food aversions.

Overall, sensory processing is vital for our ability to interact with and comprehend the environment around us.

What is a sensory food aversion?

Sensory food aversion is a condition in which a person strongly dislikes or avoids certain types of food or specific textures, aromas, tastes, or looks of food. This might be attributed to the food's sensory properties, such as texture, taste, or fragrance, which may be viewed as unpleasant, overwhelming, or painful.

Several causes can contribute to food aversions, including heredity, early food experiences, cultural or societal influences, and medical disorders. Some people may be more sensitive to specific tastes, odors, or textures, whilst others may have a higher aversion to meals connected with negative events, such as trauma.

Certain medical illnesses, such as autism spectrum disease, can cause sensory food aversions.

Overly sensitive children may avoid messy food play and meals with different textures. They frequently prefer bland flavors since strong tastes might be overwhelming. To compensate for unpleasant odors or tastes, people may smell or taste an object with a nice taste or scent, such as their clothing, to help regulate their nervous system. These children also prefer their meals to be kept at a regular temperature.

Children who are under-responsive love flavorful foods and beverages and frequently lick inedible items. They are sloppy eaters who may bite off more than their mouths can handle due to a lack of proprioception. They love both more powerful flavors and rough, crisp textures. What are the possible outcomes of sensory food aversion? Stress during mealtimes I've had an anxious eater with sensory difficulties.

I understand how difficult it may be to always worry about whether your child will eat the food you lovingly prepared. It never ends since you must feed your child every day. A nutritionist, on the other hand, can aid you in several ways. Nutritional deficiencies I hear this all the time, and the GP will not help because they are growing well along the centile.

But, as parents, you understand that it is about much more than that. If your child does not consume a variety of food categories, they risk becoming nutrient deficient. **Could it be linked to autism?** Children with autism spectrum disorder are five times more likely to experience feeding issues and are at a higher risk of nutritional deficits. Food diversity can be reduced by rejecting foods based on their flavor, smell, or texture. They often enjoy sweet or salty flavors, such as chicken nuggets, pizza, chips, or ice cream.

What can you do to help your child with a sensory food aversion?

Social modeling Keep mealtimes brief to decrease the pressure to stay at the table throughout.

Focus on the sensory qualities of food, such as color, texture, and temperature.

Let them witness you eating the items you want them to try. You can't expect kids to eat carrots unless you eat them.

Let's make eating fun again.

Mindful eating.

Encourage your children to observe and identify the food's physical properties such as size, shape, and color. In addition to food texture, warmth, aroma, and flavor.

Regular mindful eating can help alleviate food-related anxiety.

Encourage inquiry and security.

Establish a structure around meals. The timing of meals is critical.

Make an effort to stick to a consistent meal and snack plan.

Practice proper sleep hygiene. It is crucial for both mental and physical wellness. According to studies, 80% of children with autism experience sleep issues. Avoid overstimulation. Pair the new food with a favorite dish. Begin by serving a modest quantity on the side; do not force them to eat this new dish. Allow them to examine, touch, and smell the food.

Remember, there are 32 steps to eating within the six categories.

1. Toleration

2. Interaction

3. Smell

4. Touch

5. Tasting.

6. Eating.

Avoid blending more than one or two textures or temperatures into one meal. You can gradually broaden the range of textures, temperatures, and flavors over time.

Moving through textures can help with a sensory food aversion. Messy play. This might begin with dry foods and progressively increase in moisture over time. Try to complete this task outside of mealtimes.

Food preparation Encourage your child to help chop ingredients or prepare and bake their favorite biscuits. Or choose a recipe from their favorite cookbook. Find effective coping tactics when you are overstimulated.

There is no quick fix for a sensory food aversion. If sensory food aversion is interfering with a child's ability to maintain a balanced diet or affecting their quality of life, consulting with a healthcare physician or registered dietitian may be beneficial. To establish ways for overcoming the aversion and broadening the range of meals that can be consumed.

CHAPTER 5

Navigating Picky Eating Habits In Children

Parenting is full of hurdles, and genuine difficulties come while assuring your child's proper nourishment. When your child is a picky eater, it might be difficult to resolve the dinner table quandary. As a result, parents must devise effective techniques for getting their children to eat everything healthy.

Picky eating habits can be upsetting for some parents, but being patient can help you reach your goals. Understanding the developmental dynamics, avoiding power conflicts, promoting involvement, using positive language, focusing on nutritional adequacy, consistently introducing new foods, avoiding bribes, monitoring snacking patterns, establishing limits, modeling healthy behavior, creating stress-free mealtimes, and recognizing that patience is a virtue that pays off as children naturally grow out of limited

Avoiding Power Struggles: Setting the Stage for Lifelong Healthy Choices According to experts, engaging in a power struggle with a youngster over food might result in temporary gains but long-term defeats.

Establishing guidelines with a justification other than "because I'm the parent" can lay the framework for a lifetime of healthy eating.

Allow Kids to Participate: A Hands-On Approach To Mealtime Encouraging youngsters to help with meal preparation develops a sense of ownership and enhances their chances of sampling new foods. Simple household duties like draining corn or pouring milk encourage toddlers to take responsibility for their preferences.

Don't Label: Accepting Selective Eating As Normal Recognizing that infants under the age of five are often discriminating eaters, experts advise against describing them as "picky." Referring to them as "limited eaters" instead promotes a more positive attitude, avoiding pessimism.

Building On The Positives: Recognizing Comfort in Predictability Parents are urged to concentrate on the foods that their child enjoys, even if they fall within a specific range. Nutritionally, children can thrive on a few favorite foods, and growth spurts allow the opportunity to progressively introduce new foods.

Expose, Expose, Expose: Patience And Persistence In Introducing New Food A child may need to be exposed to a new cuisine 10 to 15 times before accepting it.

Parents are encouraged not to give up prematurely; consistent exposure can result in a breakthrough. It is advisable to introduce only one or two new foods per week.

Don't Bribe: Developing Healthy Habits Without External Rewards. Sweets should not be used as a reward to induce the consumption of other foods. Experts argue that the inherent reward of good nutrition is a healthy body, not extrinsic delights like chocolate cupcakes.

Beware Of Over-Snacking: Addressing Hidden Causes Over Snacking, particularly on calorie-dense meals such as chips and sweets, may lead to a child's reluctance to try new foods. Parents should make sure that snacks enhance rather than sabotage meals.

Establish "Bottom-Line Limits" for Consistency in Healthy Boundaries. Setting bottom-line limitations, such as favoring healthful foods over snacks, promotes consistency. These limitations should be appropriate, finding a balance between sound advice and flexibility.

Examine your role model: Lead by example. Parents are recommended to be cautious of their eating habits, as children frequently mimic adults.

A balanced and healthy diet in parents can have a good impact on their children's eating choices.

Defuse Mealtime: Making Food Discussions Stress-Free Separating discussions about a child's eating habits from mealtime helps alleviate stress. Experts advise postponing discussions about healthy eating for other times, such as nighttime, to avoid making every meal a potential source of conflict.

Give It Time: Growing Out Of Limiting Eating According to experts, youngsters are more likely to try new meals after the age of five. Limited eating habits are considered as a phase that many youngsters gradually overcome, highlighting the value of patience and long-term thinking.